THE ULTIMATE LEAN AND GREEN COOKBOOK FOR YOUR BREAKFAST

D1809641

50 step-by-step easy and affordable recipes for a Lean and Green food for your breakfast to start a good day and stay fit

Rachel Kim

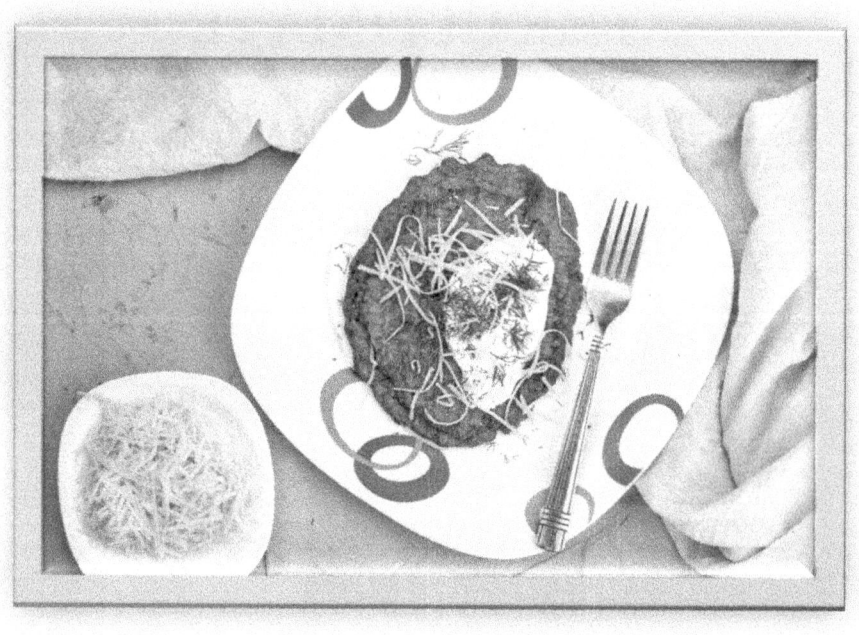

© **Copyright 2020 - All rights reserved.**

The content contained within this book may not be reproduced, duplicated or transmitted without direct written permission from the author or the publisher.

Under no circumstances will any blame or legal responsibility be held against the publisher, or author, for any damages, reparation, or monetary loss due to the information contained within this book. Either directly or indirectly.

Legal Notice:

This book is copyright protected. This book is only for personal use. You cannot amend, distribute, sell, use, quote or paraphrase any part, or the content within this book, without the consent of the author or publisher.

Disclaimer Notice:

Please note the information contained within this document is for educational and entertainment purposes only. All effort has been executed to present accurate, up to date, and reliable, complete information. No warranties of any kind are declared or implied. Readers acknowledge that the author is not engaging in the rendering of legal, financial, medical or professional advice. The content within this book has been derived from various sources. Please consult a licensed professional before attempting any techniques outlined in this book.

By reading this document, the reader agrees that under no circumstances is the author responsible for any losses, direct or indirect, which are incurred as a result of the use of information contained within this document, including, but not limited to, — errors, omissions, or inaccuracies.

Table of contents

1. Avocado Toast with Eggs

Prep Time: 15 minutes

Cook Time: 4 minutes

Serve: 4

Ingredients:

- 1 large avocado, peeled, pitted, and chopped roughly ¼ teaspoon fresh lemon juice
- Salt and ground pepper, as required 4 whole-wheat bread slices
- 4 boiled eggs, peeled and sliced

Instructions:

1. In a bowl, add the avocado and, with a fork, mash roughly.

2. Add the lemon juice, salt, and black pepper and stir to combine well. Set aside.

3. Heat a nonstick pan on meedium/high heat and toast 1 slice for about 2 minutes per side.

4. Repeat with the remaining slices.

5. Arrange the slices onto serving plates.

6. Spread the avocado mixture over each slice evenly.

7. Top each with egg slices and serve immediately.

Nutrition: Calories: 206, Fat: 13.9g, Carbohydrates: 14g, Fiber: 4.5g, Sugar: 1.4g, Protein: 9.6g

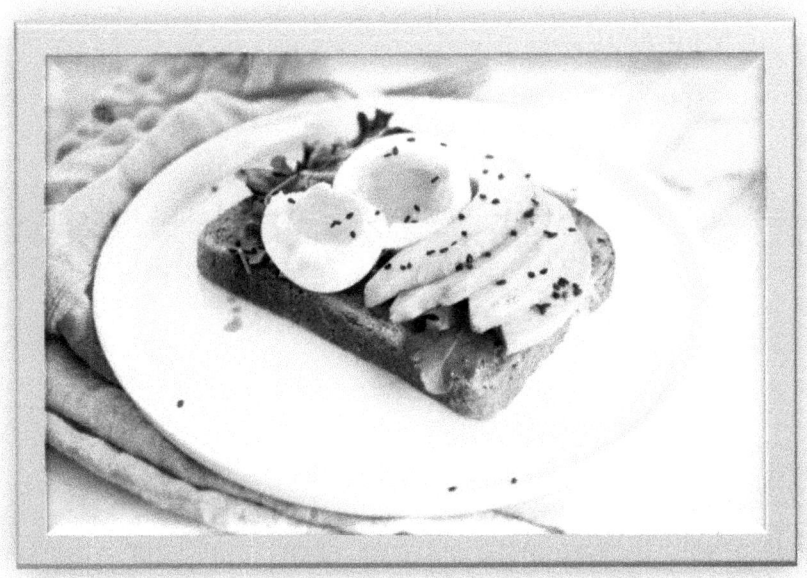

2. Toast with Egg & Asparagus

Prep Time: 10 minutes

Cook Time: 6 minutes

Serve: 2

Ingredients:

- Olive oil cooking spray
- 10 asparagus spears
- 1 teaspoon olive oil
- 2 large eggs
- 2 large sourdough bread slices, toasted Salt and ground black pepper, as required 1 teaspoon fresh rosemary leaves

Instructions:

1. Heat a griddle pan with cooking spray and heat over high heat.

2. Place the asparagus and cook for about 2-3 minutes per side.

3. Transfer the asparagus onto a plate and drizzle with a little oil.

4. Meanwhile, in a large pan, add the water and a little salt and bring to a boil over high heat.

5. Adjust the heat to low.

6. Carefully crack the eggs in the simmering water and cook for about 3 minutes.

7. With a slotted spoon, transfer the eggs onto a paper towel-lined plate to drain.

8. Divide the bread slices onto serving plates.

9. Top each slice with asparagus spears, followed by 1 egg.

10. Sprinkle with salt and black pepper and serve with the garnishing of rosemary.

Nutrition: Calories: 157, Fat: 7.5g, Carbohydrates: 14g, Fiber: 1.9g, Sugar: 1.9g, Protein: 9.8g

3. Eggs in Bell Pepper Rings

Prep Time: 10 minutes

Cook Time: 6 minutes

Serve: 2

Ingredients:

- Olive oil cooking spray
- 1 pepper, seeded and cut into 4 (¼-inch) rings
- 4 eggs
- Salt and ground black pepper, as required ¼ teaspoon dried parsley, crushed

Instructions:

1. Heat a nonstick pan with cooking spray and heat over medium heat.

2. Place 4 bell pepper rings in the pan and cook for about 2 minutes.

3. Carefully flip the rings.

4. Crack an egg of each bell pepper ring and sprinkle with salt and black pepper.

5. Cook for about 2-4 minutes or until the desired doneness of eggs.

6. Carefully transfer the bell pepper rings on serving plates and serve with the garnishing of parsley.

Nutrition: Calories: 139, Fat: 8.9g, Carbohydrates: 3.6g, Fiber: 1.1g, Sugar: 2.2g, Protein: 11.7g

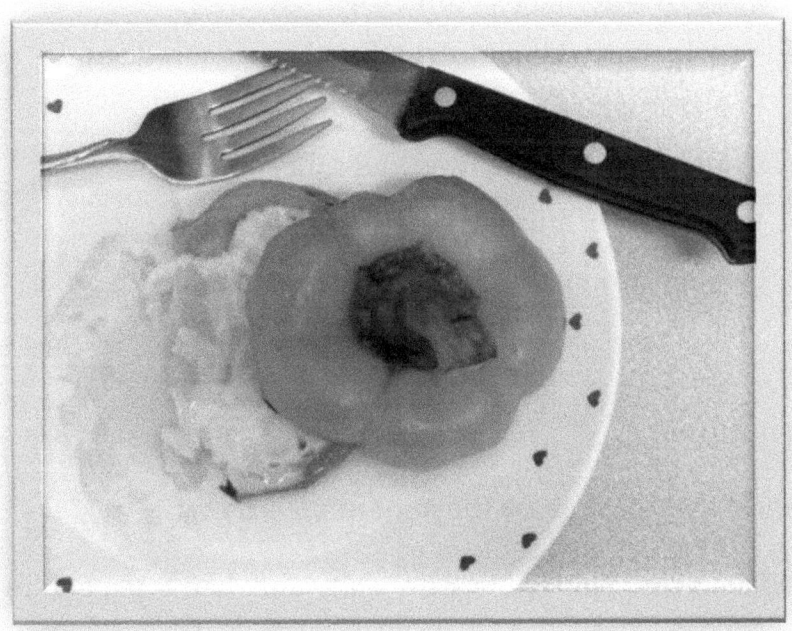

4.Spinach Waffles

Prep Time: 10 minutes

Cook Time: 20 minutes

Serve: 4

Ingredients:

- 1 large egg, beaten
- 1 cup ricotta cheese, crumbled
- ½ cup part-skim Mozzarella cheese, shredded ¼ cup low-fat Parmesan cheese, grated
- 4 ounces spinach, thawed and squeezed dry
- 1 garlic clove, minced
- Salt and ground black pepper, as required

Instructions:

1. Preheat and then grease the mini waffle iron.

2. Add cheeses, spinach, garlic, salt, and black pepper in a medium mixing bowl and mix until well blended.

3. Place ¼ of the mixture into preheated waffle iron and cook for about 4-5 minutes or until golden brown.

4. Repeat with the remaining mixture.

Nutrition: Calories: 138, Fat: 8.1g, Carbohydrates: 4.8g, Fiber: 0.6g, Sugar: 0.4g, Protein: 11.7g

5.Kale Scramble

Prep Time: 10 minutes

Cook Time: 6 minutes

Serve: 2

Ingredients:

- 4 eggs
- 1/8 teaspoon ground turmeric
- 1/8 teaspoon red pepper flakes, crushed
- Salt and ground black pepper, as required
- 1 tablespoon water
- 2 teaspoons olive oil
- 1 cup fresh kale, tough ribs removed and chopped

Instructions:

1. In a bowl, add the eggs, turmeric, red pepper flakes, salt, black pepper, and water and beat until foamy.

2. In a pan, heat the oil over meedium heat.

3. Add the egg mixture and stir to combine.

4. Immediately adjust the heat to medium-low and cook for about 1-2 minutes, stirring frequently.

5. Stir the kale in and cook for about 3-4 minutes, stirring frequently.

6.Remove from the heat and serve immediately.

Nutrition: Calories: 183, Fat: 13.4g, Carbohydrates: 4.3g, Fiber: 0.5g, Sugar: 0.7g, Protein: 12.1g

6.Tomato Scramble

Prep Time: 10 minutes

Cook Time: 5 minutes

Serve: 2

Ingredients:

- 4 eggs
- ¼ spoon red pepper flakes, crushed Salt and ground black pepper, as required ¼ cup fresh basil, chopped ½ cup tomatoes, chopped
- 1 tablespoon olive oil

Instructions:

1.Add the eggs, red pepper flakes, salt, and black pepper in a large bowl and beat well.

2.Add the basil and tomatoes and stir to combine.

3.In a non-stick pan, heat the oil over medium-high heat.

4.Add the egg mixture and cook for about 3-5 minutes, stirring continuously.

Nutrition: Calories: 195, Fat: 15.9g, Carbohydrates: 2.6g, Fiber: 0.7g, Sugar: 1.9g, Protein: 11.6g

7.Salmon & Arugula Scramble

Prep Time: 10 minutes

Cook Time: 6 minutes

Serve: 4

Ingredients:

- 6 eggs
- 2 tablespoons unsweetened almond milk Salt and ground black pepper, as required 2 tablespoons olive oil
- 4 ounces smoked salmon, cut into bite-sized chunks
- 2 cups fresh arugula, chopped finely
- 4 scallions, chopped finely

Instructions:

1.In a bowl, place the eggs, almond milk, salt, and black pepper and beat well. Set aside.

2.In a non-stick paan, heat the oil over medium heat.

3.Place the egg mixture evenly and cook for about 30 seconds without stirring.

4.Place the salmon, arugula, and scallions on top of the egg mixture evenly.

5.Adjust the heat to low and cok for about 3-5 minutes, stirring continuously.

Nutrition: Calories: 196, Fat: 15g, Carbohydrates: 2g, Fiber: 0.6g, Sugar: 1.1g, Protein: 14g

8.Apple Omelet

Prep Time: 10 minutes

Cook Time: 9 minutes

Serve: 1

Ingredients:

- 2 teaspoons olive oil, divided
- ½ of large green apple, cored and sliced thinly ¼ teaspoon ground cinnamon 1/8 teaspoon ground nutmeg
- 2 large eggs
- 1/8 teaspoon vanilla extract
- Pinch of salt

Instructions:

1.In a non-stick frying pan, heat 1 spoon of oil over medium-low heat.

2.Add the apple slices and sprinkle with nutmeg and cinnamon.

3.Cook for about 4-5 minutes, turning once halfway through.

4.Meanwhile, in a bowl, add eggs, vanilla extract, and salt and beat until fluffy.

5.Add the reemaining oil to the pan and let it heat completely.

6.Place the egg mixture over apple slices evenly and cook for about 3-4 minutes or until desired doneness.

7.Carefully turn the pan over a serving plate and immediately fold the omelet.

Nutrition: Calories: 258, Fat: 19.5g, Carbohydrates: 9g, Fiber: 1.2g, Sugar: 7g, Protein: 12.8g

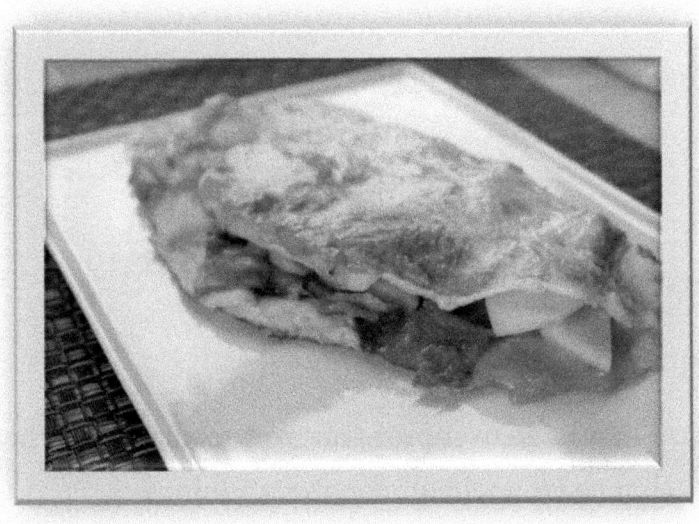

9. Veggie Omelet

Prep Time: 15 minutes

Cook Time: 15 minutes

Serve: 4

Ingredients:

- 1 teaspoon olive oil
- 2 cups fresh fennel bulb, sliced thinly
- ¼ cup canned artichoke hearts, rinsed, drained, and chopped ¼ cup green olives, pitted and chopped 1 Roma tomato, chopped
- 6 eggs
- Salt and ground black pepper, as required ½ cup goat cheese, crumbled

Instructions:

1. Preheat your oven to 325 degrees F.

2. Heat olive oil in a large ovenprof pan over medium-high heat and sauté the chopped fennel bulb for about 5 minutes.

3.Stir in the artichoke, olives, and tomato and cook for about 3 minutes.

4.Meanwhile, in a bowl, add eggs, salt, and black pepper and beat until well blended.

5.Place the egg mixture over the veggie mixture and stir to combine.

6.Cook for about 2 minutes.

7.Sprinkle with the goat cheese evenly and immediately transfer the pan into the oven.

8.Bake for approximately 5 minutes or until eggs are set completely.

9.Remove the paan from the oven and carefully transfer the omelet onto a cutting board.

10.Cut into desired sized wedges and serve.

Nutrition: Calories: 185, Fat: 12.7g, Carbohydrates: 6.3g, Fiber: 2.3g, Sugar: 1.9g, Protein: 12g

10.Mushroom & Bell Pepper Quiche

Prep Time: 25 minutes

Cook Time: 15 minutes

Serve: 4

Ingredients:

- 6 large eggs
- ½ cup unsweetened almond milk
- Salt and ground black pepper, as required ½ of onion, chopped
- ¼ cup bell pepper, seeded and chopped ¼ cup fresh mushrooms, sliced
- 1 tablespoon fresh chives, minced

Instructions:

1.Preheat your oven to 350 degrees F.

2.Lightly grease a pie dish.

3.In a bowl, add eggs, almond milk, salt, and black pepper and beat until well blended.

4.In a separate bowl, add the onion, bell pepper, and mushrooms and mix.

5.Place the egg mixture into the prepared pie dish evenly and top with vegetable mixture.

6.Sprinkle with chives evenly.

7.Bake for approximately 20-25 minutes.

8.Remove the pie-dish from the oven and set aside for about 5 minutes.

9.Cut into 4 portions and serve immediately.

Nutrition: Calories: 121, Fat: 0g, Carbohydrates: 8g, Fiber: 0.6g, Sugar: 0.1g, Protein: 10g

11.Green Veggies Quiche

Prep Time: 15 minutes

Cook Time: 20 minutes

Serve: 4

Ingredients:

- 6 eggs
- ½ cup unsweetened almond milk
- Salt and ground pepper, as required 2 cups fresh baby kale, chopped
- ½ cup bell pepper, seeded and chopped 1 scallion, chopped
- ¼ cup fresh parsley, chopped
- 1 tablespoon fresh chives, minced

Instructions:

1.Preheat your oven to 400 degrees F.

2.Lightly grease a pie dish.

3.In a bowl, add eggs, almond milk, salt, and black pepper and beat until well blended. Set aside.

4.In another bowl, add the vegetables and herbs and mix well.

5.In the bottom of the prepared pie dish, place the veggie mixture evenly and top with the egg mixture.

6.Bake for approximately 20 minutes.

7.Remove the pie-dish from the oven and set aside for about 5 minutes before slicing.

8.Cut into desired sized wedges and serve warm.

Nutrition: Calories: 123, Fat: 7.1g, Carbohydrates: 5.9g, Fiber: 1.1g, Sugar: 1.4g, Protein: 9.8g

12.Zucchini & Carrot Quiche

Prep Time: 10 minutes

Cook Time: 40 minutes

Serve: 3

Ingredients:

- 5 eggs
- Salt and ground black-pepper, as required 1 carrot, peeled and grated 1 small zucchini, shredded

Instructions:

1.Preheat your oven to 350 degrees F.

2.Lightly grease a small baking dish.

3.In a large bowl, add eggs, salt, and black pepper and beat well.

4.Add the carrot and zucchini and stir to combine.

5.Transfer the mixture into the prepared baking-dish evenly.

6.Bake for approximately 40 minutes.

7.Remove the baking-dish from the oven and set aside for about 5 minutes.

8.Cut into equal-sized wedges and serve.

Nutrition: Calories: 119, Fat: 7.4g, Carbohydrates: 3.9g, Fiber: 0.9g, Sugar: 2.2g, Protein: 9.9g

13.Pineapple Sorbet

Prep Time: 5 min

Cook Time: None

Serve: 4

Ingredients:

- cup mint, fresh

- can pineapple-chunks (1 can = 20oz. in juice, or ½ real pineapple)

Instructions:

1.Wipe the tin or cut the real pineapple and drop it in a freezer bowl (this should freeze for around 2 hours). Keep a few chunks or a loop for garnish.

2.Using a hand blender or food mixer to mix with mint when frozen (keep a few mint leaves aside as well).

3.This seems to work better if you're using fresh pineapple, then we suggest blending first and freezing afterward.

4.When nicely combined, put in bowls and garnish each with the leftover chunks and leaves.

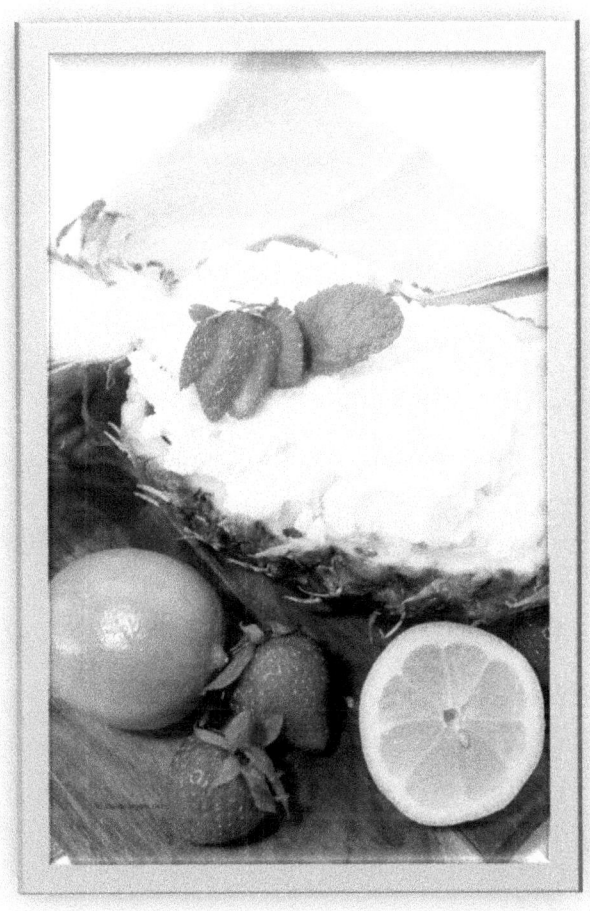

14.Bell Pepper Frittata

Prep Time: 15 minutes

Cook Time: 10 minutes

Serve: 6

Ingredients:

- 8 eggs
- 1 tablespoon fresh cilantro, chopped
- 1 tablespoon fresh basil, chopped
- ¼ spoon red pepper flakes, crushed Salt, and ground black pepper, as required 2 tablespoons olive oil
- 1 bunch scallions, chopped
- 1 cup bell pepper, seeded and sliced thinly ½ cup goat cheese, crumbled

Instructions:

1.Preheat the broiler of the oven.

2.Arrange a rack in the upper third portion of the oven.

3.In a bowl, add the eggs, fresh herbs, red pepper flakes, salt, and black pepper and beat well.

4.In an ovenproof pan, melt the butter over medium heat and sauté the scallion and bell pepper for about 1 minute.

5.Add the egg mixture over the bell pepper mixture evenly and lift the edges to let the egg mixture flow underneath and cook for about 2-3 minutes.

6.Place the cheese on top in the form of dots.

7.Now, transfer the pan under the broiler and broil for about 2-3 minutes.

8.Removee the pan from the oven and set aside for about 5 minutes before serving.

9.Cut the frittata into desired size slices and serve.

Nutrition: Calories: 167, Fat: 13g, Carbohydrates: 3.3g, Fiber: 0.6g, Sugar: 2.2g, Protein: 9.6g

15.Zucchini Frittata

Prep Time: 15 minutes

Cook Time: 19 minutes

Serve: 6

Ingredients:

- 2 tablespoons unsweetened almond milk
- 8 eggs
- Salt and ground-black pepper, as required 1 tablespoon olive oil 1 garlic clove, minced
- 2 medium zucchinis, cut into ¼-inch thick round slices ½ cup feta cheese, crumbled

Instructions:

1.Preheat your oven to 350 degrees F.

2.In a bowl, add the almond milk, eggs, salt, and black pepper and beat well. Set aside.

3.In an ovenproof-pan, heat oil over medium heat and sauté the garlic for about 1 minute.

4.Stir in the zucchini and cook for about 5 minutes.

5.Add the egg mixture and stir for about 1 minute.

6.Sprinkle the cheese on top evenly.

7.Immediately transfer the pan into the oven and bake for approximately 10-12 minutes or until eggs become set.

8.Remove the pan from the oveen and set aside to cool for about 3-5 minutes.

9.Cut into desired sized wedges and serve.

Nutrition: Calories: 149, Fat: 11g, Carbohydrates: 3.4g, Fiber: 0.8g, Sugar: 2.1g, Protein: 10g

16.Chicken & Asparagus Frittata

Prep Time: 15 minutes

Cook Time: 12 minutes

Serve: 4

Ingredients:

- ½ cup cooked chicken, chopped
- ½ cup low-fat Parmesan cheese, grated and divided 6 eggs, beaten lightly
- Salt and ground black-pepper, as required 1/3 cup boiled asparagus, chopped ¼ cup cherry tomatoes, halved

Instructions:

1.Preheat the broiler of the oven.

2.In a bowl, add ¼ cup of the Parmesan cheese, eggs, salt, and black pepper and beat until well blended.

3.In a large oven-proof pan, melt the butter over medium-high heat and cook the chicken and asparagus for about 2-3 minutes.

4.Add the egg mixture and tomatoes and stir to combine.

5.Cook for about 4-5 minutes.

6.Remove from the heeat and sprinkle with the remaining Parmesan cheese.

7.Now, transfer the pan under the broiler and broil for about 3-4 minutes or until slightly puffed.

8.Cut into desired sized wedges and serve immediately.

Nutrition: Calories: 158, Fat: 9.6g, Carbohydrates: 1.6g, Fiber: 0.4g, Sugar: 1g, Protein: 16.2g

17.Eggs with Spinach

Prep Time: 10 minutes

Cook Time: 22 minutes

Serve: 2

Ingredients:

- 6 cups fresh baby spinach
- 2-3 tablespoons water
- 4 eggs
- Salt and ground black pepper, as required 2-3 tablespoons feta cheese, crumbled

Instructions:

1.Preheat your oven to 400 degrees F.

2.Lightly grease 2 small baking dishes.

3.In a large frying-pan, add spinach and water over medium heat and cook for about 3-4 minutes.

4.Remove the frying pan from heat and drain the excess water completely.

5.Divide the spinach into prepared baking dishes evenly.

6.Carefully crack 2 eggs in each baking dish over spinach.

7.Sprinkle with salt and peppeer and top with feta cheese evenly.

8.Arrange the baking dishes onto a large cookie sheet.

9.Bake for approximately 15-18 minutes.

Nutrition: Calories: 171, Fat: 11.1g, Carbohydrates: 4.3g, Fiber: 2g, Sugar: 1.4g, Protein: 15g

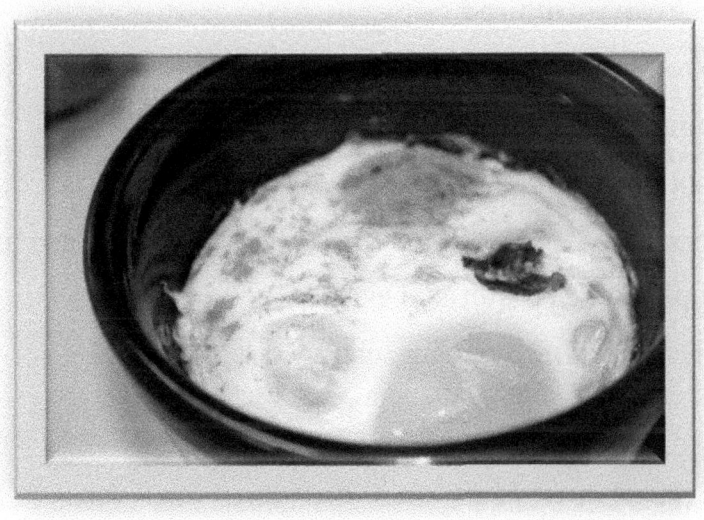

18. Eggs with Spinach & Tomatoes

Prep Time: 15 minutes

Cook Time: 25 minutes

Serve: 4

Ingredients:

- 2 tablespoons olive oil
- 1 yellow onion, chopped
- 2 garlic cloves, minced
- 1 cup tomatoes, chopped
- ½ pound fresh spinach, chopped
- 1 teaspoon ground cumin
- ¼ spoon red pepper flakes, crushed Salt, and ground black pepper, as required 4 eggs
- 2 tablespoons fresh parsley, chopped

Instructions:

1. In a non-stick pan, heeat the olive oil over medium heat and sauté the onion for about 4-5 minutes.

2. Add the garlic and sauté for approximately 1 minute.

3.Add the tomatoes, spices, salt, and black pepper and cook for about 2-3 minutes, stirring frequently.

4.Add in the spinach and cook for about 4-5 minutes.

5.Carefully crack eggs on top of spinach mixture.

6.With the lid, cover the pan and cook for about 10 minutes.

7.Serve hot with the garnishing of parsley.

Nutrition: Calories: 160, Fat: 11.9g, Carbohydrates: 7.6g, Fiber: 2.6g, Sugar: 3g, Protein: 8.1g

19.Chicken & Zucchini Muffins

Prep Time: 15 minutes

Cook Time: 15 minutes

Serve: 4

Ingredients:

- 4 eggs
- ¼ cup olive oil
- ¼ cup of water
- 1/3 cup coconut flour
- ½ teaspoon baking powder
- ¼ teaspoon salt
- ¾ cup cooked chicken, shredded
- ¾ cup zucchini, grated
- ½ cup low-fat Parmesan cheese, shredded 1 tablespoon fresh oregano, minced 1 tablespoon fresh thyme, minced
- ¼ cup low-fat cheddar cheese, grated

Instructions:

1.Preheat your oven to 400 degrees F.

2.Lightly greease 8 cups of a muffin tin.

3.In a bowl, add the eggs, oil, and water and beat until well blended.

4.Add the floour, baking powder, and salt, and mix well.

5.Add the remaining ingredients and mix until just blended.

6.Place the muffin mixture into the prepared muffin cup evenly.

7.Bake for approximately 13-15 minutes or until tops become golden brown.

8.Remove muffin tin from oven and place onto a wire rack to cool for about 10 minutes.

9.Invert the muffins onto a platter and serve warm.

Nutrition: Calories: 270, Fat: 20g, Carbohydrates: 3.5g, Fiber: 1.4g, Sugar: 0.9g, Protein: 18g

20. Turkey & Bell Pepper Muffins

Prep Time: 15 minutes

Cook Time: 20 minutes

Serve: 4

Ingredients:

- 8 eggs
- Salt and ground pepper, as required 2 tablespoons water
- 8 ounces cooked turkey meat, chopped finely
- 1 cup bell pepper, seeded and chopped
- 1 cup onion, finely chopped

Instructions:

1.Preheat your oven to 350 degrees F.

2.Grease 8 cups of a muffin tin.

3.In a bowl, add the eggs, salt, black pepper, and water and beat until well blended.

4.Add the meat, bell pepper, and onion and stir to combine.

5.Place the mixture into the prepared muffin cups evenly.

6.Bake for approximately 17,30-20,30 minutes or until golden brown.

7.Remove the muuffin tin from the oven and place onto a wire rack to cool for about 10 minutes.

8.Carefully invert the muffins onto a platter and serve warm.

Nutrition: Calories: 238, Fat: 11.7g, Carbohydrates: 4.4g, Fiber: 1g, Sugar: 2.5g, Protein: 28.2g

21. Tofu & Mushroom Muffins

Prep Time: 15 minutes

Cook Time: 30 minutes

Serve: 6

Ingredients:

- 2 teaspoons olive oil, divided
- 1½ cups fresh mushrooms, chopped
- 1 scallion, chopped
- 1 teaspoon garlic, minced
- 1 teaspoon fresh rosemary, minced Freshly ground black pepper, as required
- 1 (12.3-ounce) package lite firm silken tofu, drained ¼ cup unsweetened almond milk
- 2 tablespoons nutritional yeast
- 1 tablespoon arrowroot starch
- ¼ teaspoon ground turmeric

Instructions:

1. Preheat your oven to 375 degrees F.

2. Grease a 12 cups muffin tin.

3.In a non-stick pan, heat 1 spoon of oil over medium heat and sauté scallion and garlic for about 1 minute.

4.Add the mushrooms and sauté for about 5-7 minutes.

5.Stir in the rosemary and black pepper and remove from the heat.

6.Set aside to cool slightly.

7.In a food processor, add the tofu, remaining oil, almond milk, nutritional yeast, arrowroot starch, turmeric, and pulse until smooth.

8.Transfer the tofu mixture into a large bowl.

9.Add the mushroom mixture and gently stir to combine.

10.Move the mixture uniformly into the muffin cups that have been prepared.

11.Bake for 20-22 minutes or until it comes out clean with a toothpick inserted in the center.

12.Remove the mufin tin from the oven and place onto a wire rack to cool for about 10 minutes.

13. Invert the muffins onto the wire rack carefully.

Nutrition: Calories: 70, Fat: 3.6g, Carbohydrates: 4.3g, Fiber: 1.3g, Sugar: 1.1g, Protein: 55.7g

22.Alkaline Blueberry Spelt Pancakes

Prep Time: 6 minutes

Cook Time: 20 minutes

Serve: 3

Ingredients:

- 2 cups Spelt Flour
- 1 cup Coconut Milk
- 1/2 cup Alkaline Water
- 2 tbsps. Grapeseed Oil
- 1/2 cup Agave
- 1/2 cup Blueberries
- 1/4 tsp. Sea Moss

Instructions:

1. Mix the spelled flour, agave, grapeseed oil, hemp seeds, and sea moss in a bowl.

2. Add in 1 cup of hemp milk and alkaline water to the mixture until you get the consistency mixture you like.

3. Crimp the blueberries into the batter.

4. Heat the skillet to moderate heat, then lightly coat it with the grapeseed oil.

5. Pour the batter into the skillet, then let them cook for approximately 5 minutes on every side.

Nutrition: Calories: 203 kcal Fat: 1.4g Carbs: 41.6g Proteins: 4.8g

23.Alkaline Blueberry Muffins

Prep Time: 5 Minutes

Cook Time: 20 minutes

Serve: 3

Ingredients:

- 1 cup Coconut Milk
- 3/4 cup Spelt Flour
- 3/4 Teff Flour
- 1/2 cup Blueberries
- 1/3 cup Agave
- 1/4 cup Sea Moss Gel
- 1/2 tsp. Sea Salt
- Grapeseed Oil

Instructions:

1. Adjust the temperature of the oven to 365 degrees.

2. Grease 6 regular-size muffin cups with muffin liners.

3. In a bowl, mix sea salt, sea moss, agave, coconut milk, and flour gel until they are properly blended.

4. You then crimp in blueberries.

5. Coat the muffin pan lightly with the grapeseed oil.

6. Pour in the muffin batter.

7. Bake for at least 30 minutes until it turns golden brown.

Nutrition: Calories: 160 kcal Fat: 5g Carbs: 25g Proteins: 2g

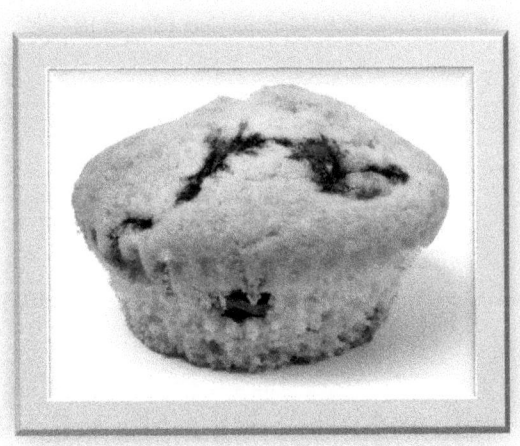

24.Crunchy Quinoa Meal

Prep Time: 5 minutes

Cook Time: 25 minutes

Serve: 2

Ingredients:

- 3 cups of coconut milk
- 1 cup rinsed quinoa
- 1/8 tsp. ground cinnamon
- 1 cup raspberry
- 1/2 cup chopped coconuts

Instructions:

1. In a saucepan, pour milk and bring to a boil over moderate heat.

2. Add the quinoa to the milk and then bring it to a boil once more.

3. You then let it simmer for at least 15 minutes on medium heat until the milk is reduced.

4. Stir in the cinnamon, then mix properly.

5. Cover it, then cook for 8 minutes until the milk is completely absorbed.

6. Add the raspberry and cook the meal for 30 seconds.

Nutrition: Calories: 271 kcal Fat: 3.7g Carbs: 54g Proteins: 6.5g

25.Coconut Pancakes

Prep Time: 5 minutes

Cook Time: 15 minutes

Serve: 4

Ingredients:

- 1 cup coconut flour
- 2 tbsps. arrowroot powder
- 1 tsp. baking powder
- 1 cup of coconut milk
- 3 tbsps. coconut oil

Instructions:

1. In a medium container, mix in all the dry ingredients.

2. Add the coconut milk and 2 tbsps. Of the coconut oil, then mix properly.

3. Drop a spoon of flour into the skillet and then swirl the pan into a smooth pancake to distribute the batter uniformly.

4. Cook it for like 3 minutes on medium heat until it becomes firm.

5. Turn the pancake to the other side, then cook it for another 2 minutes until it turns golden brown.

6. Cook the remaining pancakes in the same process.

Nutrition: Calories: 377 kcal Fat: 14.9g Carbs: 60.7g Protein: 6.4g

26. Quinoa Porridge

Prep Time: 5 minutes

Cook Time: 25 minutes

Serve: 2

Ingredients:

- 2 cups of coconut milk
- 1 cup rinsed quinoa
- 1/8 tsp. ground cinnamon
- 1 cup fresh blueberries

Instructions:

1. In a saucepan, boil the coconut milk over high heat.

2. Add the quinoa to the milk, then bring the mixture to a boil.

3. You then let it simmer for 15 minutes on medium heat until the milk is reduced.

4. Add the cinnamon, then mix it properly in the saucepan.

5. Cover the saucepan and cook for at least 8 minutes until the milk is completely absorbed.

6. Add in the blueberries, then cook for 30 more seconds.

Nutrition: Calories: 271 kcal Fat: 3.7g Carbs: 54g Protein:6.5g

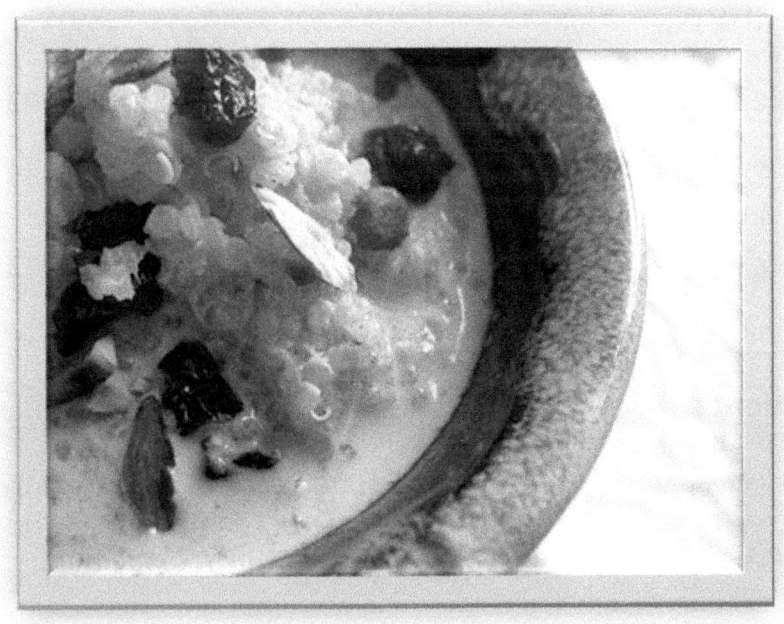

27.Amaranth Porridge

Prep Time: 5 minutes

Cook Time: 30 minutes

Serve: 2.

Ingredients:

- 2 cups of coconut milk
- 2 cups alkaline water
- 1 cup amaranth
- 2 tbsps. coconut oil
- 1 tbsp. ground cinnamon

Instructions:

1. In a saucepan, mix the milk with water, then boil the mixture.

2. You stir in the amaranth, then reduce the heat to medium.

3. Cook on medium heat and then simmer for at least 30 minutes as you occasionally stir it.

4. Turn off the heat.

5. Add in cinnamon and coconut oil, then stir.

Nutrition: Calories: 434 kcal Fat: 35g Carbs: 27g Protein: 6.7g

28.Banana Barley Porridge

Prep Time: 15 minutes

Cook Time: 5 minutes

Serve: 2

Ingredients:

- 1 cup divided unsweetened coconut milk 1 small peeled and sliced banana 1/2 cup barley
- 3 drops liquid stevia
- 1/4 cup chopped coconuts

Instructions:

1. In a bowl, properly mix barley with half of the coconut milk and stevia.

2. Cover the mixing bowl, then refrigerate for about 6 hours.

3. In a saucepan, mix the barley mixture with coconut milk.

4. Cook for about 5 minutes on moderate heat.

5. Then top it with the chopped coconuts and the banana slices.

Nutrition: Calories: 159kcal Fat: 8.4g Carbs: 19.8g Proteins: 4.6g

29.Zucchini Muffins

Prep Time: 10 minutes

Cook Time: 25 minutes

Serve: 16

Ingredients:

- 1 tbsp. ground flaxseed
- 3 tbsps. alkaline water
- 1/4 cup walnut butter
- 3 medium over-ripe bananas
- 2 small grated
- zucchinis
- 1/2 cup coconut milk
- 1 tsp. vanilla extract
- 2 cups coconut flour
- 1 tbsp. baking powder
- 1 tsp. cinnamon
- 1/4 tsp. sea salt

Instructions:

1. Tune the temperature of your oven to 375°F.

2. Grease the muffin tray with the cooking spray.

3. In a bowl, mix the flaxseed with water.

4. In a glass bowl, mash the bananas, then stir in the remaining ingredients.

5. Properly mix and then divide the mixture into the muffin tray.

6. Bake it for 25 minutes.

Nutrition: Calories: 127 kcal Fat: 6.6g Carbs: 13g Protein: 0.7g

30.Millet Porridge

Prep Time: 10 minutes

Cook Time: 20 minutes

Serve: 2

Ingredients:

- Sea salt
- 1 tbsp. finely chopped coconuts
- 1/2 cup unsweetened coconut milk
- 1/2 cup rinsed and drained millet
- 1-1/2 cups alkaline water
- 3 drops liquid stevia

Instructions:

1. Sauté the millet in a non-stick skillet for about 3 minutes.

2. Add salt and water, then stir.

3. Let the meal boil, then reduce the amount of heat.

4. Cook for 15 minutes, then add the remaining ingredients. Stir.

5. Cook the meal for 4 extra minutes.

6. Serve the meal with toping of the chopped nuts.

Nutrition: Calories: 219 kcal Fat: 4.5g Carbs: 38.2g Protein: 6.4g

31.Jackfruit Vegetable Fry

Prep Time: 5 minutes

Cook Time: 5 minutes

Serve: 6

Ingredients:

- 2 finely chopped small onions
- 2 cups finely chopped cherry tomatoes
- 1/8 tsp. ground turmeric
- 1 tbsp. olive oil
- 2 seeded and chopped red bell peppers
- 3 cups seeded and chopped firm jackfruit
- 1/8 tsp. cayenne pepper
- 2 tbsps. chopped fresh basil leaves
- Salt

Instructions:

1. In a greased skillet, sauté the onions and bell peppers for about 5 minutes.

2. Add the tomatoes, then stir.

3. Cook for 2 minutes.

4. Then add the jackfruit, cayenne pepper, salt, and turmeric.

5. Cook for about 8 minutes.

6. Garnish the meal with basil leaves.

Nutrition: Calories: 236 kcal Fat: 1.8g Carbs: 48.3g Protein: 7g

32.Zucchini Pancakes

Prep Time: 15 minutes

Cook Time: 8 minutes

Serve: 8

Ingredients:

- 12 tbsps. alkaline water
- 6 large grated zucchinis
- Sea salt
- 4 tbsps. ground Flax Seeds
- 2 tips. olive oil
- 2 finely chopped jalapeño peppers
- 1/2 cup finely chopped scallions

Instructions:

1. In a bowl, mix water and the flax seeds, then set it aside.

2. Pour oil into a large non-stick skillet, then heat it on medium heat.

3. The add the black pepper, salt, and zucchini.

4. Cook for 3 minutes, then transfer the zucchini into a large bowl.

5. Add the flaxseed and the scallion mixture, then properly mix it.

6. Preheat a griddle, then grease it lightly with the cooking spray.

7. Pour 1/4 of the zucchini mixture into the griddle, then cook for 3 minutes.

8. Flip the side carefully, then cook for 2 more minutes.

9. Repeat the procedure with the remaining mixture in batches.

Nutrition: Calories: 71 kcal Fat: 2.8g Carbs: 9.8g Protein: 3.7g

33.Squash Hash

Prep Time: 2 minutes

Cook Time: 10 minutes

Serve: 2

Ingredients:

- 1 tsp. onion powder
- 1/2 cup finely chopped onion
- 2 cups spaghetti squash
- 1/2 tsp. sea salt

Instructions:

1. Using paper towels, squeeze extra moisture from spaghetti squash.

2. Place the squash into a bowl, then add the salt, onion, and onion powder.

3. Stir properly to mix them.

4. Spray a non-stick cooking skillet with cooking spray, then place it over moderate heat.

5. Add the spaghetti squash to the pan.

6. Cook the squash for about 5 minutes.

7. Flip the hash browns using a spatula.

8. Cook for 5 minutes until the desired crispness is reached.

Nutrition: Calories: 44 kcal Fat: 0.6g Carbs: 9.7g Protein: 0.9

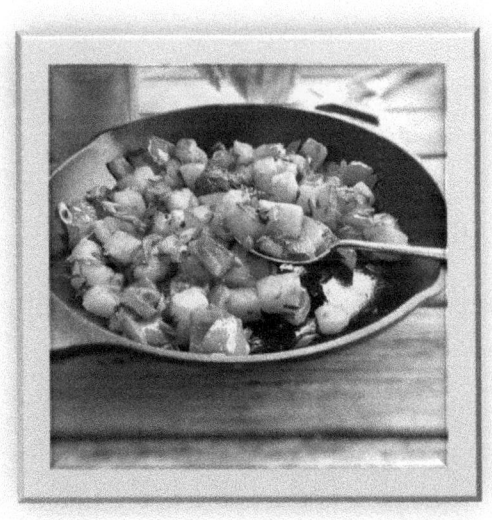

34. Hemp Seed Porridge

Prep Time: 5 minutes

Cook Time: 5 minutes

Serve: 6

Ingredients:

- 3 cups cooked hemp seed
- 1 packet Stevia
- 1 cup of coconut milk

Instructions:

1. In a saucepan, mix the rice and the coconut milk over moderate heat for about 5 minutes as you stir it constantly.

2. Take the pan out of the burner, then add it to the Stevia. Stir.

3. Serve in 6 bowls.

Nutrition: Calories: 236 kcal Fat: 1.8g Carbs: 48.3g Protein: 7g

35.Pumpkin Spice Quinoa

Prep Time: 10 minutes

Cook Time: 0 minutes

Serve: 2

Ingredients:

- 1 cup cooked quinoa
- 1 cup unsweetened coconut milk
- 1 large mashed banana
- 1/4 cup pumpkin puree
- 1 tsp. pumpkin spice
- 2 tips. chia seeds

Instructions:

1. In a container, mix all the ingredients.

2. Seal the lid, then shake the container properly to mix.

3. Refrigerate overnight.

Nutrition: Calories: 212 kcal Fat: 11.9g Carbs: 31.7g Protein: 7.3g

36.Easy, healthy Greek Salmon Salad

Prep Time: 10 minutes

Cook Time: 8 minutes

Serve: 4

Ingredients:

- ¼ cup olive oil
- 3 tablespoons red wine vinegar
- 2 tablespoons freshly crush lemon juice (from 1 lemon)
- 1 clove of garlic, chopped
- ¾ teaspoon dried oregano
- 1/2 teaspoon Kosar salt
- ¼ teaspoon fresh black pepper
- One finely chopped red onion
- A cup of cold water
- 4 (6 oz) salmon fillets, peeled
- 2 medium-sized Korean salads, such as Boston or Bibb (about 1 kilogram), broken into bite-size pieces
- 2 medium-sized tomatoes, cut into 1-inch pieces
- 1 medium English cucumber, quadrilateral and then cut into 1/2-inch pieces

- ½ cup of half-length Kalamata olives 4 oz Feta Cheese, minced (about 1 cup)

Instructions:

1. In the middle of the oven, arrange a shelf and heat to 425 degrees Fahrenheit. While the oven is warming, marinate the salmon and soften the onion (instructions below).

2. Put the olive oil, vinegar, lemon juice, garlic, oregano, salt and pepper in a large bowl, then transfer three tablespoons of vinegar large enough into a baking dish to keep all the salmon chunks in one layer. Add the salmon, lightly rotate a few times to wrap evenly in the wings. Cover the fridge. Pour the onion and water into a small bowl and set aside 10 minutes to make the onion stronger. Drain and release the liquid.

3. Discover the salmon and grill for 8 to 12 minutes until they are cooked and lightly fried. Thermometer instant-read in the middle of the thickest tab should record 120 degrees Fahrenheit to 130 degrees Fahrenheit for the rare medium or 135 degrees Fahrenheit to 145 degrees Fahrenheit. The cooking depends on the thickness of the salmon, depending on the thickest portion of the fillet. It Al depends on the salad.

4. Add the salad, tomatoes, cucumbers, olives, and red onion to the Gina Vine bowl and salt to combine. Divide into four plates or shallow bowl. When the salmon is ready, place one fillet over each salad. Sprinkle with feta and serve quickly.

Nutrition: Calories: 351 Total fat: 4g Cholesterol: 94mg Fiber: 2g Protein: 12g Sodium: 327mg

37.Mediterranean Pepper

Prep Time: 5 minutes

Cook Time: 20 minutes

Serve: 4

Ingredients:

- 1/2 teaspoon restrained oil 1/2 cup sun-dried tomatoes
- 2 cups of spinach (fresh or frozen)
- 1/2 spoon drops of zaatar spices
- 10 eggs, screaming
- 1/2 cup Feta cheese
- 1-2 tablespoons
- salt and pepper

Instructions:

1. At 350 degrees Fahrenheit, firstly preheat the oven

2. Heat a cast-iron boiler over medium heat. Add the olive oil and peas, slowly and slowly cooking until you want to release the liquid and start to brown and brown. Then, sauté the sun-dried

tomatoes with a little reserved oil, spinach and zucchini, and cook for 2-3 minutes until the spinach is crushed.

3. When the spinach has faded, pour the vegetable mixture evenly into the cast iron fish and then add the boiled eggs, turning the pan so that the eggs cover the vegetables evenly. Bake on medium heat until the eggs start about halfway through. Pour the eggs and vegetables with the spatula into the pan, leave the eggs to cook until the frittata is placed.

4. When the eggs are almost half cooked, add the Feta cheese and spoon the horseradish sauce on top and dust with salt and pepper. Remove the cast iron from the oven and place it in the middle rack in the oven. Bake until cooked on the ferrite; it will take about five minutes.

5. Bring out from the oven and let it cool slightly. For cedar, cut or square the pie and pour with a pan.

Nutrition: Calories: 311 Total fat: 4g Cholesterol: 84mg Fiber: 2g Protein: 12g Sodium: 357mg

38.Black Beans and Sweet Potato Tacos

Prep Time: 10 minutes

Cook Time: 30 minutes

Serve: 6

Ingredients:

- 1 lb. sweet potato (about 2 medium teaspoons), skin cut and cut
- into 1/2-inch pieces
- Divide into 2 tablespoons of olive oil
- 1 tablespoon Kosar salt, divided
- ¼ teaspoon fresh black pepper on large white or yellow onion, finely chopped
- 2 teaspoons of red pepper
- 1 cumin with a teaspoon
- 1 (15 oz.) can be black beans, drained and drained Cup of water
- ¼ cup freshly chopped garlic
- 12 pcs. Corn
- To serving guacamole
- Sliced cheese or feta cheese (optional)

- Wood Wedge

Instructions:

1. In the oven, set out a shelf in the middle and place to 425 degrees Fahrenheit. Set a big sheet of aluminum foil on the work surface. Collect the tortillas from the top and wrap them completely in foil. Put it aside

2. Put sweet potatoes on a small baking sheet. Mix with one tablespoon oil and sprinkle with 1/2 teaspoon salt and 1/4 teaspoon black pepper. Discard to mix and play in one layer. Fry for 20 minutes. Sprinkle the potatoes with a flat lid and set aside until a corner of the oven is clear.

3. Put the foil wrapping in the space and continue to cook for about 10 minutes until the sweet potatoes are browned and stained and the seasonings are heated. Also, cook the beans.

4. You then heat one tablespoon remaining in a large skillet over low heat. Put the onion and cook, occasionally stirring, until translucent, about 3 minutes. Mix the pepper powder, cumin, and 1/2 teaspoon salt. Add the beans and water.

5. Shield the pan and reduce the heat to low heat. Cook for 5 minutes, then slice and use the fork's back to chop the beans a

little, about half of the total. If water still remains in the vessel, stir the exposed mixture for about 30 seconds until evaporated.

6. Peel the sweet potatoes and add the cantaloupe to the black beans, and mix. If used, fill the yolk with a mixture of black beans and top with guacamole and cheese. Serve with lime wedges.

Nutrition: Calories: 251 Total fat: 4g Cholesterol: 94mg Fiber: 2g Protein: 15g Sodium: 329mg

39.Seafood Cooked from Beer

Prep Time: 30 minutes

Cook Time: 1 hour

Serve: 8

Ingredients:

Seafood:

- Canola oil for roasting
- 1/2 Cup Coarse cornmeal
- 1/2 tablespoon red pepper
- 1/4 baking soda
- 1 1/2 Cup Flour for all purposes is divided
- Kosher salt and freshly ground black pepper
- 1 12 oz can drink beer in style
- 1 code and skin without skin, cut into 8 strips
- 1 large cup (number 25/25) of peeled and spread shrimp (remaining tail)
- 16 percentiles, shake
- 1 lemon sliced with cedar wedge

- Tartar sauce, mignon, chimichurri, hot sauce, and malt vinegar, for cedar.

Sos tartar:

- 1/2 Cup Mayonnaise
- 2 teaspoons, pickled, chopped or pureed
- 1 tablespoon fresh lemon juice
- 1 tablespoon three-quarter pants
- 1 tablespoon mustard
- Kosher salt and freshly ground black pepper
- 1/2 cup Red wine vinegar
- 1 small rest, finely chopped

Kosher salt and chimichurri of freshly ground black pepper:

- 1/2 Cup Fresh parsley on a flat-leaf
- 1/4 Cup White wine vinegar
- 2 tablespoons olive oil
- 2 cloves of minced garlic
- 1 stem, seeds and mincemeat
- 1 tablespoon fresh oregano, chopped
- Sare Kosar

Instructions:

1. Heat 1 1/2-inch oil in a large Dutch oven over medium heat at 375 degrees F (deep-fried temperature with a thermometer).

2. Meanwhile, chop corn, bell pepper, baking soda, 1 cup of flour, 1/2 teaspoon salt, and 1/2 teaspoon pepper in a bowl. Add the broth and the phloem to mix.

3. Put 1/2 cup of the remaining flour in a bowl. Add salt, pepper and the fish, shrimps, shells, and lemon slices, and serve little.

4. Work several pieces at once, remove the seafood and the lemons from the flour, shake too much, drain the dough and allow the excess drops to return to the container. Carefully add the hot oil, being careful not to overload the pot. Roast golden brown and cook for 1 to 2 minutes. Transfer to a sheet of paper towel — season with salt.

5. Make the tartar sauce: mayonnaise, pickled or mixed the cloves, and pour the lemon juice, pepper, and mustard whole in a bowl. Season with Kosar salt and freshly ground pepper; feel free to add more lemon juice. Face 2/3 glass.

6. To Make a Mignonette: add red wine vinegar and finely minced mustard in a bowl. Season with Kosar salt and freshly ground pepper; allow standing for at least 30 minutes or up to 24 hours. Make 1/2 cup.

7. Make Chimichurri: Combine parsley, white wine vinegar, olive oil, garlic, jalapeño, and fresh oregano in a bowl. It is seasoned with Kosar salt. Face 2/3 glass.

8. It is served with lemon wedges, tartar sauce, mignon, chemicals, hot sauce, and malt vinegar.

Nutrition: Calories: 221 Total fat: 4g Cholesterol: 94mg Fiber: 2g Protein: 12g Sodium: 327mg

40.Crab Chicken

Prep Time: 20 minutes

Cook Time: 40 minutes

Serve: 8

Ingredients:

- Canola oil for roasting
- 1c coarse cornflour
- 1/2 Cup Flour, spoon, and surface used
- 3/4 Cup Baking powder
- 1/2 spoon
- 1/4 tablespoon
- Sare Kosar
- 2 graphic, finely chopped
- 1 tablespoon crushed peas
- Eat 8 ounces of claw crab meat (2.11 c)
- 4 oz. of Gruyère cheese, chilled (about 1 cup)
- 1 c Dough water
- 1 you tie

Instructions:

1. Heat 1 1/2-inch oil in a large Dutch oven over medium heat up to 350 degrees F (deep-fry).

2. Meanwhile, mix the cornmeal, flour, baking powder, cayenne, baking soda, and 3/4 teaspoon salt in a bowl. Add onion and onion and mix to combine. Add the crab meat and cheese and mix with a fork to combine. In the center of a well, add the butter and egg and mix to combine.

3. Spoon soup into the hot oil and be careful not to spill the pan and fry, occasionally turning until browned, 3 to 5 minutes. Transfer toa sheet of paper towel — season with salt repeat with the remaining dough.

Nutrition: Calories: 351 Total fat: 4g Cholesterol: 94mg Fiber: 2g Protein: 12g Sodium: 319mg

41.Slow Lentil Soup

Prep Time: 10 minutes

Cook Time: 20 minutes

Serve: 6

Ingredients:

- 4 cups (1 quart) of low sodium vegetable juice
- 1 (14 oz.) tomatoes can (no leak)
- 1 small, fried yellow onion
- 1 medium carrot, sliced
- 1 medium-sized celery stalk, one-piece
- 1 cup green lentils
- 1 teaspoon of olive oil, plus more for cedar
- 2 cloves of garlic, turn
- 1 teaspoon Kosar salt
- 1 teaspoon tomato paste
- 1 leaf
- 1/2 teaspoon below ground
- 1/2 teaspoon of ground coriander
- 1/4 teaspoon of smoked peppers
- 2 tablespoons red wine vinegar

- Serving options: plain yogurt, olive oil, freshly chopped parsley or coriander leaves

Instructions:

1. Put all ingredients, except vinegar, in a slow cooker for 1/3 to 2-4 quarts and mix to combine. Cover and cook in the LOW settings for about 8 hours until the lentil is tender.

2. Remove bay leaf and mix in red wine vinegar. If desired, place a pot, a drop of olive oil and fresh parsley or crushed liquid in a bowl.

Nutrition: Calories: 231 Total fat: 4g Cholesterol: 64mg Fiber: 2g Protein: 12g Sodium: 368mg

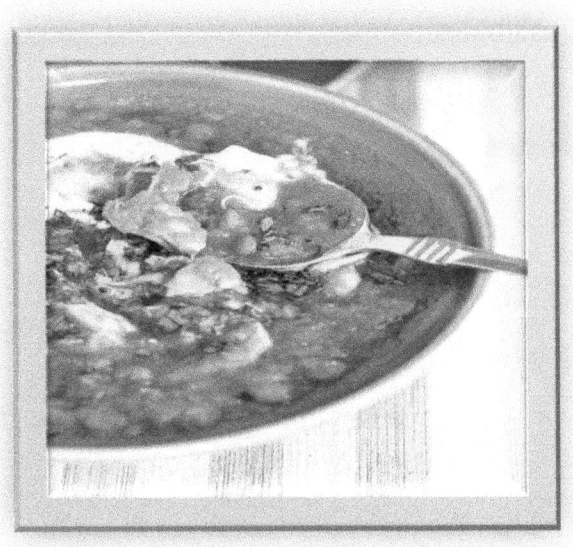

42.Light Bang Shrimp Paste

Prep Time: 10 minutes

Cook Time: 20 minutes

Serve: 4

Ingredients:

For crunchy crumbs:

- 1 tablespoon oil without butter
- Fresh cups or pancakes
- 1/8 teaspoon Kosar salt
- 1/8 teaspoon fresh black pepper
- Pepper racks
- Spend garlic powder

For shrimp pasta:

- Cooking spray
- ½ cup of Greek yogurt whole milk
- 2 tablespoons of Asian sweet pepper sauce, such as the iconic eel
- 1 teaspoon of honey
- ¼ teaspoon of garlic powder

- The juice is divided into 2 medium lemons (about 1/4 glass)
- 12 ounces of dried spaghetti
- 1 cup shrimp without skin and peeled
- 1 teaspoon Kosar salt, plus for pasta juice
- ¼ teaspoon fresh black pepper
- 1/8 teaspoon cayenne pepper
- 2 Moderated onions, sliced, sliced

Instructions:

1. Make crisp crumbs:

2. Over low heat, defrost the butter in a skillet. Add crumbs, salt, black pepper, cayenne pepper, and garlic powder. Cook while constantly stirring, until golden, crispy and fragrant. It will take 4 - 5 minutes, then put it aside.

3. Make shrimps:

4. Place a shelf in the middle of the oven and heat to 400 degrees

Fahrenheit. Cover with a lightly cooked baking sheet with cooking spray. Put it aside

5. Boil salt water in a big pot. Meanwhile, chop yogurt, pepper sauce, honey, garlic powder and half of the lemon juice in a small bowl. Put it aside

6. Add the pasta when the water boils and boil the pasta for up to 10 minutes, or as directed. Dry the shrimps and place them on a sheet of ready-made cooking. Season with salt, black pepper and coffee and mix to cook. It stretches in a uniform layer. Roast once, until the shrimps are matte and pink, 6 to 8 minutes. Pour the remaining lemon juice over the shrimps, pour over it and pour the flavored pieces onto the baking sheet.

7. Evacuate the pasta and return it to the pot. Pour into the yogurt sauce and serve until well cooked. Put shrimp and juice on a baking sheet with half of the onion and lightly add it again. Generously sprinkle each portion with a crunchy crumb and remaining onion. Serve immediately.

Nutrition: Calories: 351 Total fat: 4g Cholesterol: 94mg Fiber: 2g Protein: 12g Sodium: 327mg

43.Sweet and Smoked Salmon

Prep Time: 35 minutes

Cook Time: 1 hour

Serve: 8

Ingredients:

- 2 tablespoons light brown sugar
- 2 tablespoons smoked peppers
- 1 tablespoon shaved lemon peel
- Sare Kosar
- Freshly chopped black pepper
- Salmon fillets on the skin 1/2 kilogram

Instructions:

1. Soak a large plate (about 15 cm by 7 inches) in water for 1 to 2 hours.

2. It is heated over medium heat. Combine sugar, pepper, lemon zest, and 1/2 teaspoon of salt and pepper in a bowl. Mix the salmon with the salt and rub the mixture of spices in all parts of the meat.

3. Put the salmon on the wet plate, skin down — oven, covered, in the desired color, 25 to 28 minutes for medium.

Nutrition: Calories: 321 Total fat: 4g Cholesterol: 54mg Fiber: 2g Protein: 12g Sodium: 337mg

44.Chocolate Cherry Crunch Granola

Prep Time: 10 minutes

Cook Time: 20 minutes

Serve: 6

Ingredients:

- 3 cups rolled oats
- 2 cups assorted seeds, such as sesame, chia, sunflower, and pepitas (hulled pumpkin seeds)
- 1 cup sliced almonds
- 1 cup unsweetened coconut flakes
- 2 teaspoons vanilla extract
- 2 teaspoons ground cinnamon
- 1 teaspoon fine sea salt
- ½ cup of cocoa powder
- ½ cup pure maple syrup
- ¼ cup coconut oil or canola oil
- 1 cup dried cherries (unsweetened, if possible)
- 1 cup of chocolate chips

Instructions:

1. Preheat the oven to 350°F. Spread 2 large baking sheets with parchment paper.

2. In a large bowl, stir together the oats, seeds, almonds, and coconut. Add the vanilla, cinnamon, salt, and cocoa powder. Stir to combine.

3.Heat the maple syrup and coconut-oil in a low-heat frying pan. Pour the warm syrup and oil over the oat mixture and stir to coat. On the prepared baking sheets, spread the granola in even layers.

4. Bake for 15 to 18 minutes, scraping and mixing occasionally, then remove from the oven.

5. Put in the dried cherries and chocolate chips, then return to the oven, now turned off but still warm, and let the granola cool and dry completely.

Nutrition: Calories: 570 Total fat: 31g Cholesterol: 94mg Fiber: 2g Protein: 12g Sodium: 204mg

45. Creamy Raspberry Pomegranate Smoothie

Prep Time: 5 minutes

Cook Time: 5 minutes

Serve: 1

Ingredients:

- 1½ cups pomegranate juice
- ½ cup unsweetened coconut milk
- 1 scoop vanilla protein powder (plant-based if you need it to be dairy-free)
- 2 packed cups fresh baby spinach
- 1 cup frozen raspberries
- 1 frozen banana (see Tip)
- 1 to 2 tablespoons freshly compressed lemon juice

Instructions:

1. In a blender, combine the pomegranate juice and coconut milk. Add the protein powder and spinach. Give these a whirl to break down the spinach.

2. Add the raspberries, banana, and lemon juice, then top it off with ice. Blend until smooth and frothy.

Nutrition: Calories: 303 Total fat: 3g Cholesterol: 0mg Fiber: 2g Protein: 15g Sodium: 165mg

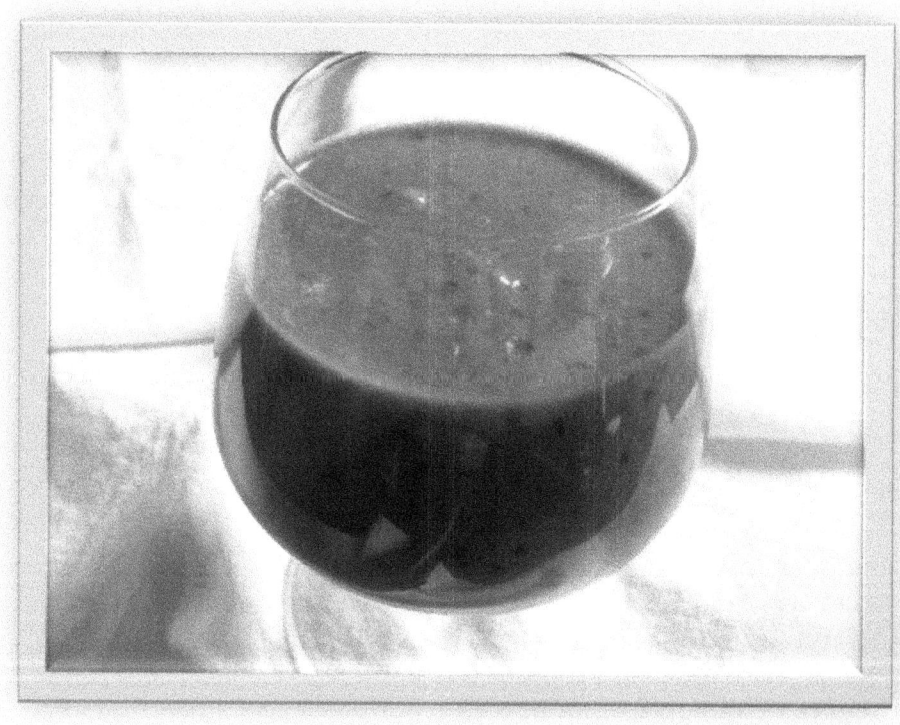

46.Mango Coconut Oatmeal

Prep Time: 5 minutes

Cook Time: 5 minutes

Serve: 2

Ingredients:

- 1½ cups water
- ½ cup 5-minute steel cut oats
- ¼ cup unsweetened canned coconut milk, plus more for serving (optional)
- 1 tablespoon pure maple syrup
- 1 teaspoon sesame seeds
- Dash ground cinnamon
- 1 mango, stripped, pitted, and divide into slices
- 1 tablespoon unsweetened coconut flakes

Instructions:

1. In a frying pan over high heat, boil water. Put the oats and lower the heat. Cook, occasionally stirring, for 5 minutes.

2. Put in the coconut milk, maple syrup, and salt to combine.

3. Get two bowls and sprinkle with the sesame seeds and cinnamon. Top with sliced mango and coconut flakes.

Nutrition: Calories: 373 Total fat: 11g Cholesterol: 0mg Fiber: 2g Protein: 12g Sodium: 167mg

47.Spiced Sweet Potato Hash with Cilantro-Lime Cream

Prep Time: 20 minutes

Cook Time: 30 minutes

Serve: 2

Ingredients:

- For the cilantro-lime cream
- 1 avocado, halved and pitted
- ¼ cup packed fresh cilantro leaves and stems
- 2 tablespoons freshly squeezed lime juice
- 1 garlic clove, peeled
- 1 teaspoon kosher salt
- ½ teaspoon ground cumin
- 2 tablespoons extra-virgin olive oil
- For the hash
- ½ teaspoon kosher salt
- 1 large sweet potato, cut into ¾-inch pieces
- 2 tablespoons extra-virgin olive oil
- 1 onion, thinly sliced
- 2 garlic cloves, crushed

- 1 red bell pepper, thinly sliced
- 1 teaspoon ground cumin
- ¼ teaspoon ground turmeric
- Pinch freshly ground black pepper
- 2 tablespoons fresh cilantro leaves, chopped
- ½ jalapeño pepper, seeded and chopped (optional)
- Hot sauce, for serving (optional)

Instructions:

1. To make the cilantro-lime cream

2. Add the avocado flesh in a food compressor. Add the cilantro, lime juice, garlic, salt, and cumin. Whirl until smooth when the processor is running slowly, softly. Taste and adjust seasonings, as needed. If there is no food processor or blender for you,, simply mash the avocado well with a fork; the results will have more texture but will still work. Cover and refrigerate until ready to serve.

3. To make the hash

4. Boil saltwater in a medium pot over high heat. Add the sweet potato and cook for about 20 minutes until tender. Drain thoroughly.

5. Over low heat, heat the olive oil. In a large skillet until it shimmers. Add the onion and sauté for about 4 minutes until translucent. Put the garlic and cook, turning, for about 30 seconds. Add the cooked sweet potato and red bell pepper. Season the hash with cumin, salt, turmeric, and pepper. For 5 to 7 minutes, Saute until the sweet potatoes are golden and the red bell pepper is soft.

6. Divide the sweet potatoes between 2 bowls and spoon the sauce over them. Scatter the cilantro and jalapeño (if using) over each and serve with hot sauce (if using).

Nutrition: Calories: 520 Total fat: 43g Cholesterol: 0mg Fiber: 2g Protein: 12g Sodium: 1719mg

48.Open-Face Egg Sandwiches with Cilantro-Jalapeño spread

Prep Time: 20 minutes

Cook Time: 10 minutes

Serve: 2

Ingredients:

For the cilantro and jalapeño spread

- 1 cup filled up fresh cilantro leaves and stems (about 1 bunch)
- 1 jalapeño pepper, seeded and roughly chopped
- ½ cup extra-virgin olive oil
- ¼ cup pepitas (hulled pumpkin seeds), raw or roasted
- 2 garlic cloves, thinly sliced
- 1 tablespoon freshly squeezed lime juice
- 1 teaspoon kosher salt

For the eggs

- 4 large eggs
- ¼ cup milk
- ¼ to ½ teaspoon kosher salt

- 2 tablespoons butter

For the sandwich

- 2 slices bread
- 1 tablespoon butter
- 1 avocado, halved, pitted and divided into slices
  Microgreens or sprouts, for garnish

Instructions:

1. To make the cilantro and jalapeño spread

2. In a food processor, combine the cilantro, jalapeño, oil, pepitas, garlic, lime juice, and salt. Whirl until smooth. Refrigerate if making in advance; otherwise, set aside.

3. To make the eggs

4. In a medium bowl, whisk the eggs, milk, and salt.

5. Dissolve the butter in a skillet over low heat, swirling to coat the pan's bottom. Pour in the whisked eggs. Cook until they begin to set then, using a heatproof spatula, push them to the sides, allowing the uncooked portions to run into the bottom of the skillet. Continue until the eggs are set.

6. To assemble the sandwiches

7. Toast the bed and spread it with butter.

8. Spread a spoonful of the cilantro-jalapeño spread on each piece of toast. Top each with scrambled eggs.

9. Arrange avocado over each sandwich and garnish with microgreens.

Nutrition: Calories: 711 Total fat: 4g Cholesterol: 54mg Fiber: 12g Protein: 12g Sodium: 327mg

49.Scrambled Eggs with Soy Sauce and Broccoli Slaw

Prep Time: 5 minutes

Cook Time: 10 minutes

Serve: 2

Ingredients:

- 1 tablespoon peanut oil, divided
- 4 large eggs
- ½ to 1 tablespoon soy sauce, tamari, or Bragg's liquid aminos
- 1 tablespoon water
- 1 cup shredded broccoli slaw or another shredded vegetable
- Kosher salt
- Chopped fresh cilantro for serving
- Hot sauce, for serving.

Instructions:

1. In a medium nonstick skillet or cast-iron skillet over medium heat, heat 2 teaspoons of peanut oil, swirling to coat the skillet.

2. In a small bowl, whip the eggs, soy sauce, and water until smooth. Pour the eggs into the pan and let the bottom set. Using a wooden spoon, spread the eggs from one side to the other a couple of times so the uncooked portions on top pool into the bottom. Cook until the eggs are set.

3. In a medium container, stir together the broccoli slaw, the remaining 1 teaspoon of peanut oil, and a salt touch. Divide the slaw between 2 plates.

4. Top with the eggs and scatter cilantro on each serving. Serve with hot sauce.

Nutrition: Calories: 222 Total fat: 4g Cholesterol: 374mg Fiber: 2g Protein: 12g Sodium: 737mg

50.Tasty Breakfast Donuts

Prep Time: 5 minutes

Cook Time: 5 minutes

Serve: 4

Ingredients:

- 43 grams' cream cheese
- 2 eggs
- 2 tablespoons almond flour
- 2 tablespoons erythritol
- 1 ½ tablespoons coconut flour
- ½ teaspoon baking powder
- ½ teaspoon vanilla extract
- 5 drops Stevia (liquid form)
- 2 strips bacon, fried until crispy

Instructions:

1. Rub coconut oil over the donut maker and turn it on.

2. Pulse all ingredients except bacon in a blender or food processor until smooth (should take around 1 minute).

3. pour batter into the donut maker, leaving 1/10 in each round for rising.

4. Leave for 3 minutes before flipping each donut. When you pierce them, leave for another 2 minutes or until the fork comes out clean.

5. Take donuts out and let cool.

6. Repeat steps 1-5 until all batter is used.

7. Crumble bacon into bits and use to top donuts.

Nutrition: Calories: 60 Fat: 5g Carbs: 1g Fiber: 0g Protein: 3g

Lightning Source UK Ltd.
Milton Keynes UK
UKHW020656110321
380169UK00012B/893